The MAGNESIUM SOLUTION
for Migraine Headaches

JAY S. COHEN, MD

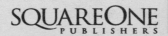
SQUAREONE
PUBLISHERS

The information and advice contained in this book are based upon
the research and the personal and professional experiences of the
author. They are not intended as a substitute for consulting with a
health care professional. The publisher and author are not respon-
sible for any adverse effects or consequences resulting from the
use of any of the suggestions, preparations, or procedures discussed in this book. All matters pertaining to your physical health
should be supervised by a health care professional. It is a sign of
wisdom, not cowardice, to seek a second or third opinion.

COVER DESIGNER: Phaedra Mastrocola
IN-HOUSE EDITOR: Amy Tecklenburg
TYPESETTER: Gary A. Rosenberg

Square One Publishers
115 Herricks Road • Garden City Park, NY 11040
516-535-2010 • 877-900-BOOK • www.squareonepublishers.com

Library of Congress Cataloging-in-Publication Data
Cohen, Jay S.
   The magnesium solution for migraine headaches : the complete
guide to using magnesium to prevent and treat migraines and
cluster headaches naturally / Jay S. Cohen.
      p. cm.
   Includes bibliographical references and index.
   ISBN 0-7570-0256-0 (pbk.)
   1. Migraine—Alternative treatment—Popular works.
2. Magnesium—Therapeutic use—Popular works. 3. Magnesium
deficiency diseases—Popular works.
   1. Migraine—drug therapy—Popular Works. 2. Cluster
Headache—drug therapy—Popular Works. 3. Magnesium—
therapeutic use—Popular Works. 4. Magnesium Deficiency—
complications—Popular Works. I. Title.
RC392.C64   2004
616.8'4912061—dc22

                                                    2004007559

Printed in the United States of America

10   9   8   7   6   5   4   3   2   1

CONTENTS

ACKNOWLEDGMENTS

I've written books before, but none with such a diverse array of people to thank. These include the pioneering members of The Erythromelalgia Association including Karl Granat, Milton Lecouter, Steve Yonker, Ray Salza, Lennia Machen, and many, many others who swapped experiences and information with me, and without whose support I would not be well or writing about magnesium today. My deepest thanks in this regard also to the world-class researchers whose knowledge helped germinate my own about erythromelalgia, allowing me to find the magnesium solution: Dr. Jill Belch of Scotland, Dr. Knut Kvernebo of Norway, Dr. Cato Mork of Denmark, Drs. Thomas Rooke and Mark Davis of the Mayo Clinic, and Dr. Haines Ely.

I would also like to thank the staff of the *Annals of Pharmacotherapy*, especially Stan Lloyd, Pharm. D.; Gene Sorkin, Pharm. D.; and Lizanne Sawyer-Kubicki, whose interest in my work led to the publication of my article on magnesium in their prestigious journal. And my special thanks to Dr. Donald Rhodes, a podiatrist and brilliant inventor, whose pioneering work in treating reflex sympathetic dystrophy led to my receiving an accurate diagnosis for the first time, without which none of this would have followed.

In my education about magnesium, many names stand out: Dr. Mildred Seelig, Dr. Burton Altura, Dr.

Chris Mende, Dr. Billie Sahley, and the Gordon Research Conferences. My knowledge has also been advanced by many doctors of integrative medicine who have shared with me their experiences in using magnesium for everyday medical disorders, such as migraine headaches and high blood pressure. Among these are: Dr. Allan Magaziner, Dr. Ron Hoffman, Dr. Jeffrey Baker, Dr. James Williams, Dr. Julian Whitaker, Dr. Alan Gaby, Dr. Alan Thal, and Dr. Dan Kalish.

My deepest personal thanks to my family and friends for their support during my long illness that helped me keep going and seeking until finding, beyond our wildest hopes and dreams, the magnesium solution. And to my medical friends who provided support and feedback and who watched in fascination as my symptoms vanished: Dr. Tony Weisenberger; Mary Weisenberger, RN; Dr. Lee Kaplan; Dr. Dennis Cook; Dede Herst, LCSW; and Dr. Roy Kaplan.

I would like to add a special acknowledgment to the thousands of doctors and other healthcare professionals who are today opening their minds beyond their heavily pharmaceutical-based sources of information and seeking knowledge about biological and natural substances that make sense scientifically and work clinically. As I've written many times, it is irrational to have two systems of medicine: mainstream and alternative. Integrative medicine, which combines the best of both, is the only medicine that makes sense. Toward this end, this book is the second of a series on natural substances and prescription drugs that I am writing to provide objective, accurate information for patients and healthcare professionals.

PREFACE

While it is accurate for me to say that magnesium stopped my migraine headaches, it also is no exaggeration for me to say that magnesium saved my life. However, it is ironic that I am the one saying it, because during my diverse medical career in general medicine, pain research, psychiatry, psychopharmacology, and now clinical pharmacology, my greatest expertise has always been prescription drugs, not natural supplements. Yet here I am writing about one of the most important natural substances for maintaining optimal health and treating a wide array of medical conditions.

I didn't learn about magnesium in medical school. Few doctors do. I learned about magnesium the hard way, twenty-eight years later. In 1995, I developed a baffling, painful, rare abnormality of the blood flow to my legs. This vascular (blood vessel) disorder with the strange name, erythromelalgia, left me bedridden for more than 3 years. I underwent all kinds of tests until I couldn't cope with being prodded and punctured any more. I tried every treatment imaginable, mainstream and alternative, to control the disorder's vicious symptoms: excessive blood flow, extreme heat, burning pain, severe swelling, and redness worse than the worst sunburn you've ever seen. I tried spinal blocks, intravenous infusions, hypnosis, biofeedback, acupuncture, hyperbaric oxygen therapy, mercury extraction from my teeth, homeopathy and herbal remedies, and many others. Most of all, I tried prescription drugs—more than 40 of them. Nothing helped at all, not even morphine. Some treatments made me worse.

Finally, at the suggestion of a Scottish researcher, Dr. Jill Belch, I tried a group of drugs I never would have considered. Calcium antagonists (calcium channel blockers) are commonly used for vascular conditions such as migraine headaches and high blood pressure, but they had also been reported to trigger my disease, and I wanted no part of any drug that could make me worse. I was already at the far end of my rope. Yet, Dr. Belch wrote that sometimes calcium antagonists actually helped erythromelalgia. She did not know why these drugs sometimes helped, and no one would have expected them to do so, but there it was. I was skeptical and scared, but I was also in terrible pain and had no other options, so I obtained a few tablets of diltiazem (Cardizem), split one into fragments, and started with a very tiny amount.

Gradually increasing the dose over the next few days and watching my body's response carefully, I noticed that my intense pain relented a little. Not much, but enough to be significant. When your pain is at level 10 (10 = maximum pain, 0 = no pain), it makes a big difference if it drops just to level 9. I wasn't even taking a quarter pill, but it was enough to help. Finally, finally, something actually helped. I was elated.

My elation was short lived. As I tried to increase the diltiazem to a more effective dose, I developed muscle spasms and overpowering malaise. Unable to raise the diltiazem enough for any consistent benefit, I switched to other drugs in the group: nifedipine (Procardia) and amlodipine (Norvasc). Both drugs provided the same enticing hint of benefit—and similar problems with unbearable side effects. I was very disappointed, yet not entirely surprised. My specific area of medical expertise is medications and their side effects. I have written medical journal articles and books on these issues, established a widely recognized website at www.MedicationSense.com, and have spoken at the highest levels. I knew that calcium antagonists cause side effects that many patients cannot tolerate. I, unfortunately, was one of them. I felt like Moses, given a vision of the promised land after years of desperation, only to be turned back in despair.

I was saved by an unlikely source. In those dark days of early 1999, somewhere from the depths of my mind a connection occurred and a question popped into my consciousness: Isn't magnesium a calcium antagonist? I don't know if this idea arose from some bit of information I absorbed long ago or from God, but magnesium is something I cannot ever remember thinking about previously. That changed quickly.

I soon learned that magnesium was an essential element for the normal activity of nerves and blood vessels, the key players in normal vascular functioning. Indeed, magnesium is the body's natural calcium antagonist, and the balance of magnesium and calcium is key to vascular health. And because magnesium is a physiological element that serves hundreds of important functions in the body, it has virtually no side effects at proper doses. The only real challenge with magnesium is getting it into your body, because most products are poorly absorbed and cause diarrhea, just like Milk of Magnesia. But once I solved this problem and was able to increase my magnesium intake, my pain quickly eased and my disorder gradually faded.

During those difficult years, I had linked up with others like me through the Erythromelalgia Association, the first and only association in the world for this very rare disorder. Soon I became a Board Member and, later, Chairman of the Medical Advisory Committee, which I remain today. As soon as I was certain of my own improvement with magnesium, I informed the other members. Not every member improved with magnesium. Erythromelalgia, like all vascular diseases, is a complex disorder with many underlying causes, so no one treatment works for everyone.

Yet many people, some disabled or bedridden for years, began to improve. Several of them traveled to San Diego to meet me. It was quite a reunion. These were people who, like me, had been severely disabled by erythromelalgia, yet there we were, meeting face-to-face for the first time after exchanging hundreds of e-mails and scores of telephone calls over the difficult years when we had pooled everything we knew in the hopes of finding something, anything to relieve the pain of a heretofore untreatable disease. Some people in our organization who were taking magnesium also reported improvements in other vascular conditions. Magnesium could help not only erythromelalgia, but also migraine headaches, high blood pressure, Raynaud's phenomenon (a condition characterized by excessive constriction of blood vessels in the fingers and toes, causing pain and spasm, in cold environments), and muscle spasms. This wasn't entirely surprising because the medical literature contains hundreds of articles on magnesium's importance for normal vascular functioning.

In February 2002, I published a scientific paper in the *Annals of Pharmacotherapy* on our group's experience with magnesium for treating erythromelalgia. In early 2004, my research was confirmed when pain specialists in Italy reported that magnesium cured an 8-year-old child with disabling erythromelalgia that hadn't responded to a variety of drugs and medical procedures.

Just after my paper on magnesium was published, I had the privilege of meeting some of the world's top researchers on magnesium. Scientists from all over the world had assembled for five days at a Gordon Research Conference to discuss one topic: magnesium. These weren't fringe scientists or alternative advocates, but academics and mainstream practitioners from the most prestigious institutions in the world. I was stunned to see so much brainpower directed toward one simple element, magnesium, which most doctors know hardly anything about and never consider for treating patients. Indeed, one of the concerns of the experts at this conference was the difficulty in getting information about magnesium into the hands of everyday practitioners. Without the resources of a drug company for advertising, free seminars, and sales representatives carrying studies and samples to doctors' offices, it is very difficult to get independent information into doctors' awareness. The magnesium researchers published their findings in medical journals, but there are hundreds of medical journals, and doctors read just a few.

Good medical care requires good information. So with my personal experience with magnesium, my knowledge of drugs and their benefits and risks, and my experience as a writer and speaker, I decided to try to bridge the gap. That's why I've written *The Magnesium Solution for Migraine Headaches*—to get the word out so that you and your doctor can consider this basic, essential element that your body needs and that you can use to help prevent or treat migraine and cluster headaches.

Most doctors are wary of supplements that come with all kinds of promises and miracle stories. They should be, and so should you. Fortunately, magnesium comes with scientific evidence that dwarfs the evidence for many top-selling prescription drugs. In writing this book, I've provided plenty of information based on scientific evidence, because it is such *evidence-based* information that your doctor will respect. The evidence for magnesium's importance in treating migraine headaches is very convincing. Yet, so few people know about it. By reading this book, you will know about it. And you can then tell other people and your doctors about magnesium, so we can provide greater relief for migraine sufferers by simply adding this safe, inexpensive, physiological element—magnesium—to the everyday prevention and treatment of this all-too-common, often disabling disorder.

Jay S. Cohen, MD

THE MAGNESIUM SOLUTION
FOR MIGRAINE HEADACHES

INTRODUCTION

A basic principle of good medical care is to use the safest medicines first when treating any disorder. Yet, mainstream medicine frequently relies on potent prescription drugs when other, safer, natural methods are all that is needed. This book is about a safe, proven-effective, natural, non-drug alternative that can be very helpful for people who get migraine and cluster headaches, that is widely available and inexpensive, that provides many benefits for the body, yet is over-looked by most doctors: magnesium.

To say that migraine and cluster headaches are painful is an understatement. Most people get tension headaches, and they assume that migraine headaches are not much different. But migraine sufferers know that migraines are a quantum beyond common tension headaches. I know, too, because in the late 1980s I began getting migraines that forced me to retreat to my bedroom, turn off the lights, stop any noise, and place an ice pack on my forehead and pray for sleep. I did not get many migraines, maybe a handful a year, but that was enough to know how truly disabling migraine headaches can be.

I do not get migraines anymore. I have not had one since 1999. I'm fortunate. Today, 25 million American adults and children—18.5 million women and 6.5 million men—suffer from migraine headaches. Cluster headaches affect another 5 million people.

Experts know that migraine and cluster headaches are among the most severe forms of pain known to humankind. Prescription medications are helpful for some people, but they are often not very helpful or cause intolerable side effects for others. I never got enough migraines to seek medical treatment, and I'm glad I did not. As magnesium caused my erythromelalgia to gradually disappear, it also had the same effect on my migraines. When I spread the word about magnesium's benefits to other members of The Erythromelalgia Association, I began receiving interesting reports about other improvements experienced by some members. Magnesium's benefits were not limited to my rare disorder, but appeared to benefit other vascular disorders as well.

In May 2001, for example, I received an e-mail from Laura, who had contacted our group on behalf of her mother, who was suffering terribly from erythromelalgia. At the end of the e-mail about her mother's status, Laura added as an afterthought:

> Incidentally, I started taking magnesium myself a couple of months ago. I was hoping it might stop my migraines which I've suffered from for seventeen years. I haven't had a migraine since—which is quite clearly, I believe, due to the magnesium. I've tried various migraine prophylactic drugs before with no improvement at all, so this is VERY good!

I asked Laura for additional details. She explained that she was a teacher, and her stress at work was very high. Laura's migraines were variable in frequency. Some weeks she would have as many as four migraines, other weeks she would have one or none. Laura had tried several prescription drugs, but none prevented the migraines and only one partially lessened the pain—if she took it quickly enough.

Laura explained: "I was prompted to start taking magnesium by the number of unsolicited comments from people who, regardless of whether magnesium helped their erythromelalgia symptoms, mentioned that their headaches or migraines had decreased or stopped." When Laura wrote to me, she had not had any migraines for several months despite the usual stresses. This was a highly unusual, excellent response, especially since so many other therapies had failed to help her. Indeed, because Laura had not responded to drugs previously, and because I never mentioned that magnesium might relieve Laura's migraines, I doubted that this was a placebo response.

Laura's next e-mail contained another surprise: "Let me tell you about my friend who gets very severe migraines." Laura wrote that he was fifty-six years old and had suffered from severe migraines his entire life. "He was often home from work sick," Laura explained. "His migraines were so bad that he was frequently incapacitated by excruciating headaches and vomiting. Several times he's been admitted to the hospital emergency department for treatment. Since starting magnesium about six weeks ago, he has only had two migraines, both of which were relatively mild and brief compared with his normal ones. He can't remember ever going for such a long time with so few migraines.

We're only a sample of two, but we're both convinced of the effectiveness of magnesium in our cases."

I would have been skeptical of Laura's reports a few years earlier, but since that time I had not only experienced my own amazing response to magnesium, but also broadened my research. I learned that since the 1960s, more than a thousand articles on magnesium had been published in medical journals. This was reassuring because when considering any treatment, whether a natural substance or a drug, you should consider the evidence. Is it convincing? Does the treatment make sense? Have studies been done? What do experts say? As you will see in this book, the evidence in all of these regards is convincing for magnesium.

Scientific evidence is important, but as every medical textbook teaches, the ultimate test is how well a treatment works for individual patients. My response to magnesium, as well as Laura's and her friend's responses, did not seem like coincidences, and the evidence supported this conclusion. Magnesium stabilizes nerve and blood vessel functioning, the two main players in vascular abnormalities such as migraine and cluster headaches, as well as in high blood pressure, Raynaud's phenomenon, and erythromelalgia. Magnesium is essential for normal vascular functioning. Blood vessels require magnesium to operate properly. Deficiencies of magnesium are common and linked to many diseases. One of these is migraine headaches (to avoid constant repetition, I will use the broad term "migraines" to include both migraine and cluster headaches unless stated otherwise).

Yet even if a treatment is effective, is it safe? As we have seen again and again in recent years, many promising drugs with outstanding research have proved ineffective for some patients and/or toxic for others, necessitating disuse or outright withdrawal. Magnesium's safety has been established over six decades. Today, magnesium is commonly used in cardiac care units for heart arrhythmias. It is used intravenously in maternity wards to treat the dangerous effects of eclampsia in pregnant women.

The unfortunate irony is that despite magnesium's long use in these medically high-risk situations, and a body of scientific evidence spanning more than half a century, few medical schools teach doctors anything about magnesium's value for everyday conditions like migraine headaches and high blood pressure. As a result, most doctors are not aware of magnesium's effectiveness for these common, often difficult-to-treat disorders. Yet, magnesium has proven its value not only in studies, but also in the offices of practitioners who have learned about it. If you go to a conference on integrative medicine and ask the brightest and best doctors about magnesium, they will relate hundreds of experiences of using magnesium with excellent results.

Nevertheless, not everyone with migraine or cluster headaches responds to magnesium. Magnesium is not a panacea. The migraine syndrome is complex, as are all vascular disorders. No single treatment works for everyone. Some migraine sufferers require prescription drugs and benefit highly from them. But why start with expensive drugs with frequent, sometimes serious side effects when safer, natural methods might do? And even when prescription drugs are needed, so too might magnesium be if the goal is to have your blood vessels function optimally. Yet, few mainstream physicians know about magnesium, so they rarely recommend it to their patients.

If you have been prescribed prescription drugs for your migraines, yet not told about magnesium, you have been denied your right of informed consent. The American Medical Association Code of Medical Ethics states that you must be given "enough information to enable an intelligent choice." You also must be told about "therapeutic alternatives consistent with good medical practice." Magnesium is certainly a therapeutic alternative consistent with good medical practice. I would argue that magnesium is a better, safer therapy that should be considered before resorting to expensive, side-effect-prone drugs.

The Magnesium Solution for Migraine Headaches is intended to provide a more balanced perspective on how to prevent and treat migraines. This book provides you and your doctor with all of the information needed to understand: why magnesium can be very helpful in preventing and/or treating migraine and cluster headaches; what you can expect from taking magnesium; and how to take magnesium successfully. This is vital information not only because, unlike drugs, magnesium has virtually no side effects at proper amounts, but the mineral also exerts hundreds of other important effects that are required for the healthy functioning of all cells and body systems. Magnesium is a key player in the normal functioning of nerves, muscles, blood vessels, bones, and the heart. So when you take magnesium, you not only may get relief from your migraine headaches, but also provide every cell and system in your body with a nutrient it needs.

CHAPTER 1

MAGNESIUM, MIGRAINES, AND CLUSTER HEADACHES

MIGRAINES: A COMMON AND SEVERE MALADY

Migraine sufferers rarely get their due. Most people get an occasional tension headache, and they assume that migraine headaches are not much different. So when Kareem Abdul-Jabbar had to leave a championship playoff game because of a migraine, basketball fans questioned his heart. But it was their hearts that should have been questioned, because the fact is that migraines are one of the most painful disorders suffered by humans.

Migraines alter people's normal functioning perhaps more than any other non-progressive disorder. The World Health Organization rates severe migraines as one of the most disabling chronic disorders in the world.[1] Oliver Sacks, the author of the popular book *Migraine*, states:

> Migraine affects a substantial minority of the population, occurs in all civilizations, and has been recognized since the dawn of recorded history. If it was

a scourge to Caesar, Paul, Kant, and Freud, it is also a daily fact of life to anonymous millions who suffer in secrecy and silence.[2]

Thomas Jefferson, Virginia Woolf, Lewis Carroll, Frederich Nietzsche, Peter Tchaikovsky, Alexander Graham Bell, Elvis Presley, and Elizabeth Taylor also endured migraines—as have tens of millions of others. Right now, in the United States, 25 million people suffer from severe migraines—18.5 million women and 6.5 million men. Over their lifetimes, about 15 percent of all people—20 percent of all women and 9 percent of all men—experience at least one migraine, and cluster headaches will affect millions more.[3,4]

Migraine pain can occur in any part of the head. It is often accompanied by nausea, and sometimes by vomiting, diarrhea, sweating, chills, tingling in the face or hands, loss of appetite, weakness, abdominal pain, fever, or intolerance to light and noise. Some migraines are preceded or accompanied by auras: double vision or spots before the eyes, impaired thinking or memory, mood disturbances, or other signs of brain dysfunction. However, most people with migraines never have aura symptoms, and they are often misdiagnosed because doctors think that aura symptoms are necessary for a migraine diagnosis. In fact, most people with migraines have never been accurately diagnosed. According to the *New England Journal of Medicine*, "Any severe and recurrent headache is most likely to be a form of migraine and to be responsive to anti-migraine therapy."[5]

Migraine attacks usually last from four to seventy-two hours. The average length is twenty-four hours, but some last two to three days. In North America, 5 percent of the entire population has at least eighteen days of migraine attacks per year. More than 3 million people have migraines one or more days each week.[6]

Migraines cause more than pain, as the *New England Journal of Medicine* describes, "Migraine has a profound effect on the well-being and general functioning of its victims, not only during the acute attacks, but also in terms of impairment of school achievement, work performance, and family/social relationships. Despite staggering social and economic costs, it remains under-diagnosed and under-treated worldwide."[7]

In some people, migraines are triggered by foods (coffee, chocolate, alcohol, spices, salt, cheese), additives, medications, changes in sleep or other biological rhythms, or the onset of menstruation. Other triggers include the scent of perfume, smoke from cigarettes or cigars, diesel or gasoline fumes, paint, bright lights or glare, stripes, blaring noise or music, or changes in the weather.[8]

BLOOD VESSELS, MIGRAINES, AND MAGNESIUM

Why does magnesium help prevent and alleviate migraines? Migraines occur when the blood vessels of the brain act erratically. Abnormal constriction and dilation of these blood vessels are the source of migraine pain, as well as the unusual visual, auditory, olfactory, or tactile sensations that more than a third of migraine sufferers experience. New theories about the origins of migraines involve heightened irritability in areas of the brain (which magnesium reduces) and serotonin imbalances, but ultimately these disturbances lead to inflammation and abnormal activity of cerebral blood vessels.

The ability of the vascular system to tighten and relax—to vasoconstrict and vasodilate—allows the body to adapt to various states such as exercise, digestion, and sleep, as well as to external circumstances such as hot or cold environments. However, sometimes the smooth muscles of the arteries constrict or dilate abnormally, and vascular disorders such as migraines, high blood pressure, Raynaud's phenomenon, and erythromelalgia occur. Together, these conditions affect more than 80 million Americans and 900 million people worldwide.

What influences the relaxing and tightening of the tiny smooth muscles lining the blood vessels? Many factors, but foremost among them is the mineral magnesium. Actually, the balance of magnesium and another mineral, calcium, in and around the muscle cells lining the arteries is a primary determinant of their state of relaxation and constriction. Calcium tends to make muscles constrict, whereas magnesium causes them to relax. Thus, when excess calcium flows into the muscle cells lining the arteries, constriction occurs.

There is a whole group of drugs, the calcium antagonists (calcium channel blockers) that doctors prescribe to block the flow of calcium into vascular muscle cells and thereby promote blood vessel relaxation. In fact, in the year 2000, doctors wrote more than 95 million prescriptions for calcium antagonists including top-sellers amlodipine (Norvasc), nifedipine

(Procardia), diltiazem (Cardizem, Tiazac), and others, at a total cost of over $4.5 billion.[9] These drugs are not only costly, but have many side effects such as dizziness, flushing, palpitations, fatigue, nausea, abdominal pain, tiredness, and swollen legs. Side effects like these cause millions of people to quit treatment, just as I quit taking diltiazem, nifedipine, and amlodipine for my erythromelalgia.

The body uses a natural mechanism to block blood vessel constriction and to maintain normal blood vessel functioning. It uses the element magnesium. Magnesium blocks calcium's influx into vascular smooth muscle cells. By blocking the influx of calcium into vascular smooth muscle cells, magnesium regulates blood vessel tone. That is why for decades experts have called magnesium the body's "natural calcium blocker."[10,11,12]

In 1961, Drs. Burton and Bella Altura, working at the State University of New York Health Science Center at Brooklyn, noticed that when vascular smooth muscle was deficient in magnesium, the tiny muscles went into spasm. The contraction could be relieved by replenishing magnesium. "In 1961, everybody was investigating calcium," Burton Altura told me. "We wondered why no one was looking at magnesium, too. So we decided to include magnesium in our tests. We were so surprised and excited by our findings, we did not believe it. We waited five or six years, after repeating our tests hundreds of times, before trying to publish anything."[13]

For over four decades, the Alturas have conducted more studies on magnesium's actions in the body and its role in more medical conditions, including hypertension, than any other research group. In a 1985 article titled "Calcium antagonist properties of magnesium: implications for antimigraine actions," the Alturas described how low magnesium levels in peripheral, coronary, and cerebral blood vessels in animals caused spasm-like responses. Increasing the magnesium produced relaxation of these arteries. The Alturas proposed that magnesium deficiencies might underlie the occurrence of migraines because magnesium:

- Stabilizes blood vessel membranes

- Inhibits blood vessel contraction that occurs in response to chemicals (serotonin, prostaglandins, norepinephrine) released in the early phase of the migraine cascade

- Inhibits the clumping of platelets

- Reduces the synthesis and release of inflammatory mediators

- Directly relaxes blood vessel tone

All of these benefits make magnesium an effective anti-migraine therapy. Indeed, magnesium is an ideal first choice because it serves these very same functions naturally in normal human systems. Magnesium is not a synthetic drug with all kinds of adverse effects, but nature's natural vascular relaxant in human and animal systems. Thus it is not surprising that the Alturas found that "in certain areas of Africa and Japan where the dietary level of magnesium is high, the incidence of migraine is among the lowest in the world."[14]

By 1998, the role of magnesium in migraines and other headaches was attracting wider recognition. "Magnesium deficiency appears to be a common denominator in all leading theories of migraine pathogenesis," Dr. Alexander Mauskop and Dr. Burton Altura wrote. "The importance of magnesium in the pathogenesis of migraine headaches is clearly established by a large number of clinical and experimental studies."[15] Other experts agreed. Dr. K.M. Welch, of the Department of Neurology, Henry Ford Health Sciences Center, Detroit, wrote, "An increasing body of evidence supports a role for systemic and brain magnesium deficiency in migraine sufferers."[16]

Dr. Sherry Rogers, a respected allergist and leading proponent of complementary medicine, has written extensively about magnesium's benefits for many disorders caused by abnormal muscle constriction. "A trial of magnesium is indicated for any spastic condition. In order for a muscle to contract, it needs calcium. In order to relax it needs magnesium. Many people have spastic conditions that smack of magnesium deficiency. One of the commonest symptoms of magnesium deficient patients are back and neck pain."[17] And migraines.

Magnesium's beneficial effects on migraines may also arise from its direct effects on nerve tissue. Some experts believe that migraine headaches result from excessive nerve excitability in the brain, which builds up and spreads, releasing inflammatory substances that cause pain. Magnesium reduces nerve excitability and inhibits its spread. Magnesium also calms pain receptors. When I took magnesium for my erythromelalgia, the first change I noticed was a reduction in pain, which occurred weeks before the vascular changes became evident.

MAGNESIUM—THE ESSENTIAL ELEMENT FOR NORMAL BODY FUNCTIONING

Magnesium is a mineral that is essential for the normal functioning of the human body. Magnesium plays a key role in more than 300 different enzymatic reactions that take place within all of the body's cells. Magnesium is a necessary element in just about every step of the pathway by which cells create energy for their many activities.

Magnesium has a relaxing effect on the central nervous system and tempers the actions of the sympathetic nervous system. Magnesium is essential for cells to maintain proper balances of other minerals such as potassium, sodium, and calcium. When cells are deficient in magnesium, this balance is disrupted, and cells lose potassium and are flooded with calcium and sodium.[18] In the smooth muscle cells of the blood vessels, this sets the stage for the constriction and subsequent dilation of the migraine cascade.

Magnesium is also necessary for the proper metabolism of zinc, iron, copper, and phosphorus, as well as for calcium, potassium, and sodium. Within cells, magnesium is essential for regulating many biochemical activities, including the proper metabolism of glucose (blood sugar). Magnesium is essential for normal growth, nerve transmission, wound healing, muscle contraction, and the proper conduction of electrical impulses that govern the functioning of the heart. This mineral is required for the metabolism of essential fatty acids and many vitamins. Magnesium is an essential element in bone formation and bone resiliency, and it helps to prevent kidney stones. In addition, according to Dr. Sherry Rogers, "Magnesium is one mineral that is in just about every single phase of the detox pathway."[19]

One of America's best-known doctors of integrative medicine, Dr. Julian Whitaker, writes:

> I often refer to magnesium as my favorite mineral, and with good reason. Magnesium has a known therapy effect on the heart and cardiovascular system; is involved in at least 325 enzymatic reactions throughout the body; helps maintain potassium in the cells; and is vitally important to healing wounds, muscular function, sleep, growth, and healthy pregnancy. Research has overwhelmingly demonstrated the critical relationship between low levels of magnesium and cardiovascular disease.[20]

Dr. Rogers does not hesitate to add, "Magnesium is definitely the king of minerals. It has solved more 'incurable' and 'mysterious symptoms' than any other mineral I have observed in 31 years."[21]

MAGNESIUM VS. PRESCRIPTION DRUGS FOR MIGRAINE HEADACHES

The medical treatment of migraines has improved over the last several decades. Many people have been helped by prescription drugs, but many people have not, and side effects are frequent and can be serious. Magnesium offers an alternative that is not only natural to your body, but is also as effective as many prescription drugs. Magnesium is also far less expensive.

Drugs for Acute Migraines

The most prescribed drugs for treating acute migraines are the *triptans:* Amerge (naratriptan), Frova (frovatriptan), Imitrex (sumatriptan), Maxalt (rizatriptan), Replax (eletriptan), and Zomig (zolmitriptan). Triptans are the first drugs specifically designed to alleviate migraine headaches, which they do by blocking serotonin receptors in blood vessels in the brain. This results in a reduction in artery dilation and inflammation. For most people, triptans are more effective than earlier migraine drugs, and they can be taken orally or, for fast relief, by injection or as a nasal spray.

Triptan drugs are specifically used for halting acute migraine attacks as they are developing. Triptans work very well for some people, but not for others. Triptans cannot be used for preventing migraines, they are very expensive, use is limited, and side effects are frequent and sometimes serious.[22,23]

The package inserts of triptans contain long lists of potential side effects, including: chest pain, chest pressure, dizziness, nausea, weakness, diarrhea, abdominal pain, flushing, drowsiness, shortness of breath, ringing in the ears, tingling, muscle tightness, or sensations of warmth in the head, neck, chest, or limbs. Moreover, triptans are known to cause spasm of coronary arteries and have been directly linked to angina, heart attacks, cardiac arrhythmias, strokes, and sudden death.[24] Indeed, the U.S. Food and Drug Administration (FDA) requires that package inserts of triptan drugs carry this warning: "Serious adverse cardiac events, including acute myocardial infarction, life-threatening disturbances of cardiac rhythm, and death have been reported within a few hours of administration of 5-HT1 agonists [triptans]."[25]

The overuse of triptans can also cause problems. According to a recent study, the overuse of medications for acute migraines, including triptans, can lead to the development of chronic daily headaches.[26] Moreover, many people cannot take triptans because the drugs are contraindicated for those with high blood pressure, elevated cholesterol, diabetes, or obesity. Triptans are also contraindicated for smokers, menopausal women, and people with strong family histories of coronary artery disease. That includes a lot of people. In addition, males over age 40 are advised to have a thorough cardiovascular evaluation before receiving triptans,[27] although there are reports of people who had normal cardiovascular testing yet sustained serious cardiac reactions after taking triptans.[28]

In order to be effective, triptans must be taken quickly, when migraine pain is just emerging. Once a migraine has been established, triptans are not usually helpful.[29]

Another problem with triptans involves the injectable form of Imitrex, which is widely used to stop acute migraines. With the autoinjector, the standard dose of injectable Imitrex is 6 milligrams. This one-size-fits-all dosage is strong because it is designed to cover a broad population of patients, yet injectable Imitrex is also associated with the greatest risk of serious cardiovascular reactions.

There is a way to reduce this risk, although most doctors are not aware of it. If you look at the package insert for injectable Imitrex, you will see a large table showing that just 2 milligrams of injectable Imitrex—67 percent less than the standard dose of 6 milligrams—provides relief for about 43 percent of migraine sufferers. Just 3 milligrams—50 percent less medication—helps 60 percent of migraine patients. In other words, the majority of patients using injectable Imitrex for acute migraines can get relief with 50–67 percent less medication than the standard one-size-fits-all dosage. This is very important because triptans' side effects are dose-related: the stronger the dose, the more frequent and severe the reactions. Using a lower dose can reduce your risk of having a serious adverse effect.

If you use injectable Imitrex, get a package insert from your pharmacist or copy it from the *Physicians' Desk Reference*.[30] Ask your doctor to take a look at the package insert and discuss whether it might be worthwhile to try a lower dose of injectable Imitrex. Better yet, ask about switching to the oral or nasal forms of the drug, which have better safety profiles. If you are taking another type of triptan, including oral triptans, it is still wise to always use the lowest effective dose. However, do not make any changes to your drug or dosage without your doctor's guidance.

These problems notwithstanding, triptan drugs are sometimes a godsend for people with severe migraines. For those who do not obtain a positive response from triptans, magnesium can help. In a 1998 study of people who did not respond satisfactorily to Imitrex, 50 percent obtained a much better response to the drug after taking magnesium supplements. The dose of magnesium in this study was low (250 milligrams daily), so the use of higher magnesium doses might provide even better results.[31] In fact, by using magnesium and/or other non-drug therapies discussed in subsequent chapters, you may be able to reduce or eliminate your need for prescription antimigraine drugs.

Other drugs are also used for acute migraines. One emergency room expert I know highly recommends intravenous Compazine (prochlorperazine) given with an intramuscular injection of Benadryl (diphenhydramine). Unfortunately, intravenous Compazine has been difficult to obtain recently. Another emergency physician who has treated many patients with acute migraines recommends intravenous Toradol (ketorolac) and Reglan (metaclorpramide). These are ideas you can pass along to your doctor. Other drugs used for halting acute migraines are ergot derivatives such as dihydroergotamine (DHE) and an ergotamine-caffeine combination marketed as Cafergot. All of these drugs come with long lists of side effects.

Drugs for Preventing Migraines

For preventing migraines, the anti-seizure drug Topamax (topiramate) has received considerable attention of late, although Topamax is far more expensive than magnesium and not as effective or safe. In a 2002 study, Topamax helped about 38 percent of chronic migraine sufferers, yet 58 percent of the subjects developed side effects.[32] In a large randomized, double blind, placebo-controlled study published in 2004, partial improvement in migraine frequency and severity was obtained by 39 percent of patients taking 50 milligrams per day of Topamax, 49 percent taking 100 milligrams, and 47 percent taking 200 milligrams. Compared with the effectiveness of magnesium, these numbers are not impressive. But Topamax's side effects are impressive: in the 100 milligrams group, 50 percent developed nerve irritation or pain, 14 percent experienced fatigue, 11 percent had diarrhea, 11 percent experienced reduced sensation, 11 percent had impaired memory, 10 percent had nausea. These are large numbers, and some side effects were serious. Overall, 27 percent of patients in this group quit treatment because of intolerable side effects.[33] That is a very high discontinuance rate, yet not surprising considering the frequency of adverse effects. For some people, the cure was obviously worse than the disease. But this does not prevent the drug industry or media from trying to make Topamax sound like a miracle drug for migraines.

In fact, memory problems with Topamax can be considerable. In one study, the doctors began jokingly calling the drug "Dopeamax." One observer noted, "A writer said a revision that should have taken her an hour took three hours. A pianist had trouble renumbering pieces. A graduate student had to read the same page over and over."[34] This is not so funny when people think they are getting Alzheimer's disease and doctors, unaware of Topamax's tendencies, deny that the drug is the cause.

So although Topamax can help some people with migraines, it comes with substantial risks—far more risks (and cost) than magnesium. Moreover, the long-term effects of using Topamax for migraines are not known, whereas it is well known that magnesium can provide not only migraine relief, but also vital benefits in hundreds of other ways to every cell in your body. If you and your doctor are considering using Topamax, it is recommended that you start with a low dose and, if necessary, increase the dose very gradually.[35]

You should also be aware that serious, new side effects continue to be discovered with Topamax including more than one hundred reported cases of glaucoma, which can cause permanent damage to the eyes. This discovery necessitated a new warning in the Topamax package insert.[36,37] Topamax has also been associated with an imbalance of acid-base metabolism known as metabolic acidosis, which can be life threatening. According to the Public Citizen Health Research Group, a serious degree of metabolic acidosis occurred in 11 percent of Topamax users.[38] As a result, the manufacturer now recommends repeated monitoring of serum bicarbonate levels.

Other drugs for preventing migraines include beta blockers such as propranolol (Inderal) and atenolol (Tenormin), calcium antagonists such as verapamil (Calan, Isoptin), anti-seizure drugs such as gabapentin (Neurontin) and divalproex (Depakote), opiates, barbiturates, anti-inflammatory drugs, drugs affecting blood vessels, and SSRI antidepressants (Zoloft, Paxil, Prozac, and others). Tricyclic antidepressants are also used, including amitriptyline (Elavil), imipramine (Tofranil), and nortriptyline (Pamelor), which is the least side-effect prone of these.

These drugs are sometimes helpful, sometimes not—and they all can cause side effects. For example: amitriptyline commonly causes weight gain and bothersome constipation; divalproex can cause nausea or dizziness; propranolol and atenolol can cause fatigue; and the frequent use of aspirin or anti-inflammatory drugs can cause stomach pain or gastric bleeding. Doctors may consider these types of side effects "minor," but patients experiencing such adverse effects do not. Medication side effects are the reason that millions of people quit treatment for many serious medical disorders.

Prescription Drugs: Satisfactory Migraine Therapy Remains Elusive

For millions of people, the mainstream medical approach to migraine and cluster headaches is clearly less than optimal. A 1996 article in the medical journal *Headache* stated: "Only about one third of all headache patients are fully satisfied with treatments currently available."[39] In 2001, migraine expert Alexander Mauskop, MD, wrote:

> Despite the new drugs, we're still in pain. Twenty-five million Americans still dread the onset of the next migraine, lose time from work, must beg off personal and family chores, and must tell friends that they can't make it today. We just don't have a drug that can reliably and safely prevent migraines from striking.[40]

In 2003, Dr. Isadore Rosenfeld, a practicing physician and well-known television commentator, concurred, "Although there are several medications available [for treating migraines], there is a lot of room for improvement."[41]

Indeed, a 2004 article underwritten by a drug company and published in *JAMA* (*Journal of the American Medical Association*) acknowledged that "even among patients who are treated, less than one third report consistently effective results with their current pharmacologic regimens."[42]

All of the drugs discussed above have their uses, but none is effective in a large percentage of migraine patients. Individual responses to all migraine drugs vary considerably. Vascular diseases are complex because many factors influence blood vessel activity. This is why no one treatment works for high blood pressure or erythromelalgia—or migraine or cluster headaches. As most migraine patients know, it is a trial-and-error process to find the best treatments at the right dose for you. Again, do not make any changes to your medications or dosages without your doctor's guidance.

On the positive side, if you look at the results of studies, the effectiveness of magnesium and other non-drug therapies discussed in the next chapter compares favorably with prescription anti-migraine drugs. And magnesium and other non-drug therapies are safer and much less expensive. I have no quarrel with the use of prescription drugs for people who need them, but I disagree with the mainstream medical approach of using drugs without even considering safer, cheaper, equally effective non-drug alternatives—especially a scientifically-proven alternative like magnesium.

CHAPTER 2

MAGNESIUM DEFICIENCY AND MIGRAINE HEADACHES

THE MOST COMMON MINERAL DEFICIENCY

In 1900, the average American diet provided about 450 milligrams of magnesium a day. In 2000, the average diet provided only 200 to 225 milligrams daily. The U.S. Recommended Daily Allowance (RDA) of magnesium is 320 milligrams per day for adult women and 420 milligrams for adult men (see Table 2.1). This means that while most Americans in 1900 were getting adequate dietary magnesium, today as many as 80 percent of Americans are magnesium deficient.[1,2] Similar deficiencies exist in all Western countries. A survey conducted in France in the mid 1990s found that 72 percent of men and 77 percent of women got less than the RDA of magnesium in their diets.[3] Magnesium deficiencies may be even more prevalent if, as some experts state, the RDA of magnesium is too low and the daily intake should actually be 500 milligrams.

Dr. Alan Gaby, one of the pioneers in the alternative medicine movement, writes: "Magnesium deficiency is one of the most common nutritional problems

Table 2.1. U.S. Recommended Dietary Allowance (RDA) for Magnesium

Different ages, genders, and situations require different daily allowances of magnesium. Stress may increase the amount needed. Some experts believe these allowances are too low. Note that the amounts listed represent milligrams (mg).

Age	Men	Women	Pregnancy	Lactating
14–18	410 mg	360 mg	400 mg	360 mg
19–30	400 mg	310 mg	350 mg	310 mg
31 or older	420 mg	320 mg	360 mg	320 mg

in the industrialized world today." He adds that while no single vitamin or mineral can cure all of the problems people sustain, "nevertheless, magnesium so often makes a difference in our lives that it deserves special attention. For millions of Americans, correcting magnesium deficiency could be one of the most important steps on the road back to health."[4]

There are many reasons that magnesium deficiencies are much more common today, despite the fact that Americans eat healthier and have many more food choices than their 1900 counterparts. Some of these reasons are:

- Agricultural fertilizers often contain inadequate amounts of magnesium.

- Accelerated growth techniques in the fields reduce the amount of time for magnesium fixation in plants.

- Refining methods often reduce the magnesium content of foods.

- Boiling vegetables causes loss of magnesium.

- Soft drinks and other popular beverages contain large amounts of phosphates, which interfere with magnesium absorption.

- High-fat diets reduce magnesium absorption.

- The increased amount of calcium that Americans get in foods and supplements reduces the absorption, and increases the kidney excretion, of magnesium.

- Consumption of large amounts of salt, coffee, and/ or alcohol can interfere with magnesium absorption or cause magnesium loss from the body.

- Some medications cause magnesium loss: diuretics, which are prescribed for hypertension and congestive heart failure; digitalis; antibiotics such as gentamicin and amphotericin; cancer drugs such as cisplatin; and immunosuppressive drugs that are used to prevent the rejection of a transplanted organ following surgery.

- Most people just do not eat enough magnesium-rich foods: green leafy vegetables, legumes, beans, nuts, soybeans and whole soy products, unprocessed cereals, and unrefined grains.

- Many people take multivitamin or multimineral supplements, but these rarely contain enough magnesium to offset dietary deficiencies. Also, the magnesium contained in many supplements is of poor quality and poorly absorbed.

- The processing of most municipal water and bottled water causes their magnesium contents to be very low.

The result is that, day after day, year after year, people are getting inadequate amounts of magnesium in their diets and, consequently, magnesium deficiencies are widespread. Yet, magnesium is essential for the normal functioning of cells and body systems, especially the vascular and nervous systems, so it is not surprising that neurovascular disorders such as migraine headaches, high blood pressure, and Raynaud's phenomenon are also widespread. This is why, of all the nutritional and non-drug methods that people can adopt to prevent and treat migraine headaches, magnesium supplementation ranks first. Yet, few people—and fewer doctors—know this.

THE EVIDENCE FOR MAGNESIUM IN THE PREVENTION OF MIGRAINE HEADACHES

In a 1991 study in Italy, twenty women with long histories of migraines during menstruation were given magnesium. Preliminary blood tests revealed that the migraine sufferers had much lower levels of magnesium in their white blood cells than people without migraine histories. Taking just 360 milligrams per day of magnesium, the women reported a marked and rapid improvement in the frequency, severity, and duration of migraine attacks. In the magnesium group, pain scores dropped from an average of 93 to 30 after just two months, and then down to 10 after four months (significantly superior to the placebo group). The researchers concluded:

> These findings demonstrate that menstrual migraine patients have intracellular magnesium deficiency

and indicate that oral magnesium supplementation improves peri-menstrual migraine with a restoration of intracellular content of magnesium. Magnesium supplementation has proven to be better than placebo, thus providing evidence of a specific pharmacological effect.[5]

However, scientific progress is rarely linear, and these promising results were refuted in a 1996 study conducted in Germany, Austria, and Switzerland, using 250 milligrams of magnesium twice daily.[6] Yet, the lack of improvement may have been due to poor absorption of magnesium, for 46 percent of patients reported side effects such as diarrhea. Without good absorption, magnesium does not work.

In another study, other European researchers gave 600 milligrams per day of magnesium to eighty-one migraine sufferers. Within three months, the frequency of migraine attacks diminished on average by 42 percent, far superior to the 16 percent improvement in the placebo group. Indeed, the people taking magnesium also reported much less reliance on other drugs for pain—a reliable sign of improvement. The authors concluded, "High-dose oral magnesium appears to be effective in migraine prophylaxis."[7]

THE EVIDENCE FOR MAGNESIUM IN THE TREATMENT OF ACUTE MIGRAINE HEADACHES

Stopping acute migraines, once they have started, is difficult. Even the most powerful drugs, the triptans, have to be started quickly upon signs of onset to provide good results. Magnesium offers a safer, effective alternative—a proven alternative.

In 1995, researchers gave 1 gram of magnesium sulfate intravenously to forty people (37 women, 3 men) having acute migraines. Thirty-five subjects (87.5 percent) obtained substantial improvement in their migraine pain. Nine obtained complete relief. The benefit lasted at least twenty-four hours for twenty-one of these thirty-five responders, a marked improvement because these people's previous migraine attacks lasted forty hours on average.[8]

A year later, these researchers published another study. Using even larger amounts of up to 3 grams of intravenous magnesium sulfate, "complete elimination of pain was observed in 80% of the patients within 15 minutes of infusion of magnesium sulfate." Some patients obtained relief lasting forty-eight hours. When the migraines returned, they typically occurred after the ionized serum magnesium levels again dropped below normal, thus further substantiating the link between migraines and serum ionized magnesium.[9] In a few patients, the magnesium infusions provided spectacular results. The youngest patient, a 14-year-old girl, had obtained no relief previously from Tylenol, Motrin, Relafen, antihistamines, or physical therapy. Yet, a single infusion of magnesium sulfate produced remission of her migraines that lasted at least five months, from the time of the study until the doctors wrote their article.

The results of these researchers were remarkable. But were they too good to be true? Independent confirmation was needed. In 2001, doctors in Turkey published their results from giving 1 gram of intravenous magnesium sulfate to fifteen people suffering severe acute migraines. Another fifteen sufferers were given a placebo intravenously. In the magnesium group, thirteen people (87 percent) had a prompt cessation of pain, and the other two obtained partial improvement. In all of the magnesium recipients, accompanying symptoms such as nausea, irritability, and intolerance of light and sound disappeared. In comparison, only one person in the placebo group noted any improvement.[10]

The doctors then treated the placebo group members with intravenous magnesium. Fourteen (93 percent) of them obtained complete pain relief, and the fifteenth obtained partial relief. All of their accompanying symptoms disappeared, too. The authors concluded: "Our results show that 1 gram of intravenous magnesium sulfate is an efficient, safe, and well-tolerated drug in the treatment of migraine attacks."[11]

Confirmation has come from other sources, too. Doctors of alternative medicine have long known about magnesium's effectiveness. Dr. Joseph Mercola offers the following information about magnesium at his popular website:

> I find that intravenous magnesium aborts well over 75% of headaches. The magnesium causes the blood vessels to dilate and makes the person very warm, depending on how fast the magnesium is pushed. I usually use 1500 mg for the average adult. This is far safer, more effective, and less expensive.[12]

But not everyone agrees. One emergency room doctor told me, "Magnesium hasn't worked well for my acute migraine patients." Another ER doctor reports that magnesium sulfate (usually 2 grams) helps about 25 percent of patients if the migraine is caught early. After twenty-four hours, any treatment will be less effective. Still, he sends people home with magnesium to prevent further attacks.

Many alternative doctors report the best results with the Myers Cocktail: an intravenous infusion containing magnesium plus vitamins and minerals. See "Treating Acute Migraines With Magnesium" on page 45 for further details.

WHY MAGNESIUM DEFICIENCIES ARE NOT IDENTIFIED OR TREATED

Magnesium researcher Dr. R. Whang writes:

> Magnesium depletion may represent the most frequently unrecognized electrolyte abnormality in clinical practice today. . . . There appears to be as much as an 85%-90% shortfall in clinical recognition of abnormal serum magnesium. . . . The role of magnesium in cellular function, both in health and disease, remains largely unknown to [medical] clinicians.[13]

The fact that humans can become deficient in magnesium was not discovered until 1956. Yet in the many decades since, only a small portion of the mainstream medical community and the general public has become aware of the prevalence of magnesium deficiencies and their impact on health. Why? The training of most medical doctors does not focus on magnesium. If doctors do not know about magnesium deficiencies, they cannot diagnose them or teach others about them. So, although a small, dedicated group of researchers around the world continues to conduct studies and hold conferences, spreading the word about magnesium has been difficult. This is not likely to change without funding from the National Institutes of Health or a foundation to subsidize the effort.

"Physicians are a lot less knowledgeable about magnesium than [they are about] calcium," Dr. Christian W. Mende, an expert on vascular functioning, has told me. "More studies on magnesium such as by the National Institutes of Health are needed for prevention and treatment of magnesium-related diseases. Research on magnesium could have as major an impact on public health as many other items the NIH is studying."[14]

The main reason that magnesium deficiency is not widely recognized is the lack of a readily available, reliable test for the condition. Today, most medical laboratories measure the total serum (blood) magnesium. This usually is not helpful because even if a person is severely deficient in magnesium, the body keeps the blood level of magnesium normal by pulling the mineral out of cells and bone. A person can have a major magnesium deficiency, yet still have a serum magnesium level that is normal. Incidentally, the same is true for calcium; thus osteoporosis is not diagnosed by a blood test, but by measuring bone density.

For decades, scientists have searched for a simple test to identify magnesium deficiencies. This has not been easy because less than 1 percent of the body's total magnesium is contained in the blood, whereas about 55 percent resides in bones, 26 percent in muscles, and 18 percent in the other tissues. Developing a test that can accurately reflect magnesium levels in the tissues has been a challenge.

The traditional test for measuring magnesium deficiencies is the magnesium loading test. Two grams of magnesium are injected intravenously or intramuscularly (intramuscular injections can be painful), and you must collect your urine over the next twenty-four hours. This is not wildly popular among patients. Yet, the test is highly accurate because people with adequate magnesium stores in their body will excrete most of the injected magnesium. People without adequate magnesium will excrete only a small portion.

The standard is that people who excrete more than 80 percent of the injected magnesium are not magnesium deficient, whereas people who excrete less than 80 percent are magnesium deficient. However, some people's genetics make them unable to retain magnesium even when they are severely deficient. Thus, with the magnesium loading test, these magnesium wasters will excrete most of the injected magnesium, and their test results will be read as normal, whereas in fact they have severe magnesium deficiencies.

More recently, Drs. Burton and Bella Altura and others have developed a test that measures the ionized (electrically charged) fraction of magnesium in the blood, rather than measuring the total serum magnesium. They call it the IMg2+ test. With acute migraine patients, they have often found "that ionized serum magnesium is low, though total magnesium is within the normal range."[15] With children experiencing post-traumatic headaches, 67 percent had low ionized serum magnesium levels, although their total serum magnesium levels were normal.[16] However, this test is not widely available, although it can be obtained by contacting Drs. Burton and Bella Altura, Department of Physiology—Box 31, SUNY Downstate Medical Center at Brooklyn, 450 Clarkson Avenue, Brooklyn, NY 11203-2056 (telephone 718-270-2194, fax 718-270-3103).

Another reliable test, known commercially as Exatest, measures the total magnesium taken from a swab of cells from your inner cheek or under your tongue. The laboratory, Intracellular Diagnostics, will send a kit to your doctor, who will smear the cells onto a slide. The laboratory uses energy-dispersive analysis to measure the level of magnesium and other minerals within the cells. This test may be covered by Medicare and other insurers. Check with Intracellular Diagnostics Inc., 553 Pilgrim Drive #B, Foster City, CA 94404, (telephone 650-349-5233), www.exatest.com.

A test that measures the level of free magnesium in red blood cells is sometimes used by doctors who practice integrative medicine. This test is available through laboratories such practitioners use.

These new tests offer promising possibilities, yet the fact is that until an accurate magnesium test is as easy to get and covered by medical insurers as other blood tests, magnesium deficiencies will continue to go undiagnosed and untreated. The fault for this lies not only with the absence of a convenient test, but first and foremost with inadequate medical education and medical practices that are overly wedded to the drug industry, which spends billions to keep doctors focused on prescription drugs, not natural substances.

Doctors who are aware of the importance of magnesium for maintaining health and treating vascular diseases will find ways around today's limitations in magnesium testing. Some doctors order the tests listed above.

On the other hand, Dr. Mende uses the standard magnesium blood test at his disposal, which is inexpensive, although not highly accurate at identifying people with magnesium deficiencies. "Still, I catch many patients with low magnesium," Dr. Mende told me.[17] He prescribes magnesium not only for people whom the test identifies as having low magnesium levels, but also for those with magnesium levels in the bottom third of the normal range.

This is not a bad approach. Experts believe that the "normal range" of the total serum magnesium test is so broad that almost everyone falls into it, yet people whose levels are in the lower end of the normal range are probably magnesium deficient. For the most accurate results, the test should be taken after fasting (in the morning before eating), and the result must be adjusted if the level of serum albumin (a type of blood protein) is abnormal. Even with these imprecise guidelines, the total serum magnesium test can identify some magnesium deficiencies.

Nevertheless, if you or your doctor has access to more accurate tests, you should use them. When these more accurate tests become widely available, testing for magnesium status will become as routine as testing people's calcium levels. The result will be a much greater recognition of magnesium deficiency, which is a truly widespread problem. Then, treatment with magnesium—which is safe, effective, and inexpensive—might finally become a standard for preventing and treating migraine headaches, high blood pressure, Raynaud's phenomenon, and other cardiovascular disorders.

CHAPTER 3

MAGNESIUM DEFICIENCIES IN MIGRAINE-PRONE POPULATIONS

WOMEN, MIGRAINES, AND MAGNESIUM

"Migraine has been labeled a 'woman's disease' because it is three times more common in women than men," read a 1998 article in *Women and Health*, "and the attacks tend to be more severe and disabling among women."[1] The statistics are indeed daunting. Twenty percent of women—versus 9 percent of men—will have at least one migraine during their lifetime. In any given year, 15–18 percent of women—versus 6 percent of men—get at least one migraine headache.[2]

The higher incidences of migraines among women seem to be related to their shifting hormone levels, especially around menstruation. Before puberty and after menopause, women have a similar migraine incidence as men. Many women experience their first migraine with the onset of menstruation, the use of birth control pills, or during pregnancy. Birth control pills can be harmful or helpful, triggering migraines in some women, improving migraines in others, and having no effect either way in other women. Also, a connection exists between premenstrual syndrome (PMS) and migraines. Thirty to sixty percent of menstruating women get PMS, which includes headaches, irritability, depression, bloating, breast tenderness, and weight gain. And as in the case of migraines, many women who get PMS also have low levels of magnesium.

Magnesium can be helpful not only for migraines, but also for PMS symptoms and menstrual pain. Chris Mende, MD, a highly respected hypertension specialist and magnesium expert, has prescribed magnesium with positive results to women with PMS symptoms or menstrual pain.[3]

Unfortunately, some women run an increased risk of magnesium deficiency because of the widespread use of calcium supplements to prevent osteoporosis. Magnesium and other minerals are also essential for maintaining healthy bone, yet calcium supplements can block magnesium absorption and increase magnesium excretion. Therefore, women taking calcium supplements should also take magnesium. Unfortunately, mainstream doctors rarely suggest this.

CHILDREN, MIGRAINES, AND MAGNESIUM

Migraine headaches in children are prevalent, often debilitating, and frequently misdiagnosed. Thirty percent of migraine sufferers have their first attack before the age of ten. Adolescents and young adults have the highest frequency of migraines.

Migraines in children usually develop without any warning signs. In contrast to adults, headache pain is often bilateral. The duration of migraines is usually more brief in children, lasting a few hours. Pain is often the only symptom, but nausea, vomiting, dizziness, fever, or sensitivity to light, sound, or odors can occur. Sometimes symptoms such as nausea or abdominal pain can occur without headaches, which makes diagnosing the migraine difficult. When these symptoms occur repeatedly, a migraine-like syndrome should be considered. Like adult sufferers, children with migraines usually want to lie down in a quiet room and sleep.

In a 1993 study in Italy, forty children with recurrent pain (25 with migraines, 12 with recurrent abdominal pain, 3 with fever from no obvious cause) were given 122–366 milligrams of magnesium daily. Six months later, 77.5 percent of the children had obtained a good response and 10 percent had achieved a partial response.[4] Subsequent studies have confirmed these results. In a four-year, double-blind, placebo-controlled study published in 2000 that involved children with at least one migraine per week, children in the placebo group improved initially but then worsened again, whereas children receiving magnesium showed gradual but continuous reductions in the number and severity of migraine symptoms.[5] In addition, a 2001 study found that the majority of children with post-traumatic headaches had magnesium deficiencies.[6]

MEN, CLUSTER HEADACHES, AND MAGNESIUM

Whereas women get more migraines than men, cluster headaches afflict men far more often than women. The duration of cluster headaches—approximately 30–90 minutes—may be briefer than migraines, but cluster headaches can occur several times a day, or sometimes every day for weeks or months.

Like migraine headaches, cluster headaches arise from changes in the brain and its blood vessels, but cluster headaches emerge from a lower part of the brain. Cluster headaches are almost always one-sided. They usually start behind an eye, and the pain is often described as piercing or burning. The eye can become teary or bloodshot, and the nostril on the same side may feel congested or runny. Some people with cluster headaches prefer to move around, rather than lying still in a dark, quiet room, as migraine sufferers do.

Magnesium can help cluster headaches. In one study of people with various types of headaches, the cluster sufferers had the lowest levels of ionized serum magnesium.[7] The results of two other studies showed that magnesium was highly effective for treating cluster headaches.[8,9]

CHAPTER 4

HOW TO USE MAGNESIUM TO HELP PREVENT AND TREAT MIGRAINE AND CLUSTER HEADACHES

MAGNESIUM: A NUTRIENT AND A MEDICATION

According to Dr. Burton Altura, those people with magnesium deficiencies generally get the greatest benefit from using magnesium for migraines. Dr. Altura states:

> Fifty percent of all migraine sufferers have magnesium deficiencies. Treatment with magnesium provides quick relief that lasts months. Of the other 50% who are not magnesium deficient, 25% still respond, which we believe is a placebo response. Other types of headaches respond similarly including tension headaches and post-traumatic headaches. The potential of the discoveries about magnesium for headaches is staggering.[1]

Fifty percent of migraine sufferers is approximately

12.5 million people (not to mention the millions more with cluster headaches). If magnesium can help this many people, it will be the most successful—and the safest and most economical—migraine therapy ever.

But Dr. Altura's numbers may underestimate the potential of magnesium for migraines. Whether or not you have a documented magnesium deficiency, magnesium may help you. Remember, in the studies using intravenous magnesium for acute migraines, 80–90 percent of patients improved with magnesium treatment. The number would be far less if only the people with documented magnesium deficiencies had responded. Why did so many more people experience improvement? Because magnesium is more than an essential nutrient. At higher doses, magnesium is a pharmacologically active substance. At higher doses, magnesium acts like a drug with clearly defined effects on the blood vessels, brain, heart, and other systems throughout the body. If a person with normal levels of magnesium is given high doses of magnesium, he or she will still experience its pharmacologic effects.

For example, if a woman who is pregnant develops eclampsia, a dangerous complication characterized by severe hypertension and a high risk of seizures, her doctor will immediately treat her with large doses of magnesium administered intravenously. The doctor will not worry whether the woman has a magnesium deficiency. Magnesium is the standard treatment because it reduces blood pressure and calms an excited nervous system quickly and safely.

Similarly, high-dose magnesium may be beneficial even for migraine sufferers who do not have magnesium deficiencies or who do not know whether they have magnesium deficiencies or not. Indeed, I did not measure my magnesium level before trying magnesium. It never occurred to me to do so. Now, after taking substantial doses of magnesium every day for years, I am certainly not magnesium deficient, but I still need magnesium. The magnesium keeps my erythromelalgia in remission, and if I discontinue the magnesium or reduce the dosage too much, my symptoms start to return. This is because magnesium has both nutritive and, at higher doses, pharmacologic effects.

Dr. Altura is correct in that the evidence of magnesium's benefits for migraines is stronger with people with magnesium deficiencies. People with documented magnesium deficiencies do have the greatest likelihood of responding well to magnesium. But this does not mean that others cannot respond, too.

Dr. Allan Magaziner, President of the American College for the Advancement of Medicine and medical director of the Magaziner Center for Wellness and Anti-Aging in Cherry Hill, NJ, orders magnesium levels on many of his patients. Yet, he told me, "Even if the test is normal, I still use magnesium. Even in people without low magnesium tests, magnesium still can have a therapeutic effect."[2]

TREATING ACUTE MIGRAINES WITH MAGNESIUM

Acute migraines require immediate treatment. Fortunately for migraine sufferers, the studies in the "Evidence" section (Chapter 2) are impressive: with 1–3 grams of magnesium sulfate intravenously, 80–90 percent of patients obtained significant, rapid relief of migraines. Unfortunately, few mainstream physicians know about these studies because most of their information comes from the drug companies—and drug companies do not push products that cannot be patented.

At the same time, among doctors using magnesium for acute migraines, the feedback has been mixed. As with any therapy, some patients respond, some do not. To obtain better results, many alternative doctors use the Myers Cocktail, which consists of magnesium chloride, calcium gluconate, B-vitamin complex, vitamin C, soluble B_{12} (hydroxocobalamin), pantothenic acid (Dexpanthenol), and pyrodoxine. Mixed in 10–20 milliliters of sterile water, the infusions are given slowly. Many patients experience warmth during infusions. Seniors, frail individuals, and people with low blood pressure tolerate less magnesium and should be started with lower doses. Specific information about doses and methods can be easily found on the Internet by searching for "Myers Cocktail" or "Myers' Cocktail."

Dr. Magaziner is an advocate of this approach, and states, "If people come in with an acute migraine, sometimes I will suggest an intravenous approach and break the migraine cycle right then."[3] Dr. Alan Gaby has written extensively about the Myers Cocktail, and reports: "I have found that a combination of magnesium, calcium, B-vitamins, and vitamin C, given intravenously, can often relieve a migraine attack within one or two minutes."[4]

Intravenous therapy works fast, but for most people it is inconvenient to have to rush to the doctor's office or to an emergency room every time a migraine looms. Unfortunately, few studies have been conducted using magnesium orally for acute migraines. My research on using high-dose oral magnesium for erythromelalgia is one of the few that addresses these issues.[5] Some people in my survey take several grams of magnesium a day, and such doses would probably also be effective for acute migraines, but further study is needed.

Dr. Rogers, the only other doctor who has written about oral magnesium for acute migraines, states, "Many folks take 200 mg of magnesium every 30 minutes at the start of a migraine (stop at 800 mg) to abort it."[6] However, this treatment is intensive and is not advised for everyone, so it should always be done with your doctor's supervision. People using liquid forms of magnesium should start with less, because liquid magnesium is more rapidly and completely absorbed than magnesium tablets.

Of course, the best treatment for acute migraine or cluster headaches is to prevent them from developing in the first place. This is very possible, and magnesium can play a central role.

PREVENTING MIGRAINE HEADACHES WITH MAGNESIUM AND OTHER NON-DRUG THERAPIES

In addition to magnesium, there are other natural, nondrug therapies that can be useful in the prevention of migraine headaches. These include riboflavin, feverfew, butterbur, SAMe, and combination therapies.

Magnesium

The scientific studies in the "Evidence" section show that magnesium can be very effective for preventing migraines. The RDA doses of 320–420 milligrams daily are sufficient for some people, but many people require higher doses. Dr. Allan Magaziner usually starts with 400 milligrams per day, but some people require 400 milligrams twice daily. Dr. Magaziner states, "Magnesium has so many beneficial effects, often patients will see other things improve such as muscle aches, general fatigue, and sleep. I find magnesium to be a very safe substance."[7]

Dr. Julian Whitaker routinely places patients on a daily regimen of 500 milligrams of magnesium and 1,000 milligrams of calcium. For people with migraines, he uses 800–1,000 milligrams of magnesium daily. He adds, "Don't hold your breath waiting for your doctor to tell you about the preventive and therapeutic value of magnesium. Start supplementing [at RDA levels; for higher levels, work with your doctor] with this indispensable mineral today."[8] Dr. Chris Mende, a mainstream physician, also recommends magnesium. "Magnesium supplementation is not 100% effective, but makes a major improvement. And it is so safe."[9]

The improvement can occur quickly, but sometimes it takes longer. It is very difficult to force magnesium into cells. In contrast, calcium will rush in to them. Thus, cells must work to get magnesium inside and then use the magnesium to block excess calcium. People differ in how quickly their cells assimilate magnesium and, of course, in the degree of their magnesium deficiencies. Some benefit from taking magnesium is usually seen within days or weeks, but the full effect may take a month or two. People with severe magnesium deficiencies may see increasing improvement over three to six months.

Dr. Alexander Mauskop has used magnesium intravenously not only for treating acute migraines, but also to actually prevent migraines from occurring. The rationale is that intravenous therapy is more effective in attaining high levels of magnesium in cells. Administering one intravenous treatment a month, Dr. Mauskop was able to prevent migraines for many patients (and to prevent some women from getting PMS, too).[10]

Riboflavin (Vitamin B$_2$)

This vitamin has a variety of roles in the body that range from assisting the cells to extract energy from protein, carbohydrates, and fat to aiding the production of red blood cells. The basis for riboflavin's effects on migraine headaches is not known, but research studies and clinical experience indicate that riboflavin works.

In a study published in 1994, researchers gave large doses of 400 milligrams per day of riboflavin for more than three months to forty-nine migraine sufferers. By the end of the study, both the severity and frequency of the subjects' migraines had decreased by more than two-thirds.[11] Impressed, the researchers conducted a follow-up study to see whether the results could be confirmed. Published in 1998, this double-blind study involved fifty-five people with migraines who received either riboflavin or placebo. After three months, about two-thirds of the people in the riboflavin group experienced a 50 percent or greater reduction in the frequency of migraine attacks and the number of days lost from work due to migraines. These results were significantly superior to those in the placebo group.[12] The best results were seen in the final month of the study.

No one knows why 400 milligrams per day of riboflavin, a very large dose, is needed to obtain benefit. Perhaps this amount is required to overcome riboflavin deficiencies. Yet, many foods contain riboflavin, and serious deficiency is uncommon. Still, a large percentage of the population gets inadequate amounts of riboflavin from their diets, so maybe even mild deficiencies must be overcome in order for riboflavin to work. This would explain why it usually takes a few months for riboflavin to have an effect on migraine headaches.

Riboflavin taken with magnesium is even more effective. Dr. Mauskop states, "Although the results with riboflavin alone are not as impressive as seen with magnesium, the combination of the vitamin and the mineral is potentially strong. You need to take megadoses of riboflavin, 400 mg, and should be prepared to wait two or three months to enjoy the benefits."[13]

Taking megadoses of riboflavin is usually safe because the kidneys excrete excess amounts of the vitamin. However, if you have impaired kidney function or are elderly, check with your doctor.

Feverfew

The herb feverfew was reported as helping to relieve headaches as early as the seventeenth century. Studies of feverfew published in the last thirty years have supported this by demonstrating reductions in the frequency, severity, and duration of migraines.

In a double-blind, placebo-controlled study published in *Lancet* in 1988, seventy-two migraine patients were given feverfew. The results showed a significant reduction in the frequency and severity of headaches.[14] A study published in 1985 examined feverfew's effect in preventing migraines in a group of seventeen migraine patients already taking feverfew. In this double-blind, placebo-controlled study, eight subjects continued to receive feverfew while nine received placebo. Over time, the members of the feverfew group reported less frequent and less severe migraines than those receiving placebo.[15] "Feverfew has been tested in five double-blind studies," Dr. Mauskop states. "There is a clear trend showing that it is better than placebo, which means it has definite benefits."[16]

The basis of feverfew's ability to prevent migraines is not known. Researchers speculate that feverfew may reduce arterial inflammation or exert effects on serotonin or histamine, factors involved in the development of many migraines. Feverfew is approved in Britain and Canada for treating migraines.[17] Like riboflavin, it may take a month or two for feverfew to work. Feverfew can inhibit clotting, so it should be avoided in people with bleeding disorders or taking anticoagulants. If you use aspirin regularly, ask your doctor about taking feverfew.

Other Supplements and Combination Therapies

To varying degrees, studies or clinical experience have

shown the following substances to be helpful for preventing migraine headaches: butterbur, SAMe (S-adenosyl-L-methionine), tryptophan, 5-HTP (5-hydroxytryptophan), coenzyme Q_{10}, glucosamine, and high doses of fish oils.[18,19] In Europe, butterbur is frequently used for preventing migraines, and high doses of melatonin are used for cluster headaches.[20]

Combination therapies are widely used for preventing migraine headaches. The most commonly used combination products contain magnesium, riboflavin, and feverfew. Dr. Mauskop recommends 300–400 milligrams of magnesium, plus 400 milligrams of riboflavin and 100 milligrams of feverfew daily. In his informative book *What Your Doctor May Not Tell You About Migraines*, Dr. Mauskop writes: "In most cases, the results are nothing short of amazing."[21] Indeed, the guidelines of the American Academy of Neurology for preventing migraines cite magnesium, riboflavin, and feverfew.[22]

Doctors of integrative medicine often employ similar combinations. "We get a good 50% resolution in the duration, intensity, and frequency of migraines," Dr. Magaziner says of combination therapy. "The duration and intensity of their headaches are much less."

Several companies make products with magnesium, feverfew, and riboflavin or B-vitamins, usually taken twice daily. Vitamin or health food stores carry products with this combination. Some doctors add other supplements to the mix. Dr. Whitaker includes 2–6 grams of a fish oil supplement daily.[23] Dr. Alan Gaby recommends magnesium, riboflavin, feverfew, and 6–15 grams per day of a fish oil concentrate.[24]

WHERE TO BEGIN

My philosophy about supplements is no different than about medications: the best treatment is the least amount that works. I recommend starting with magnesium and seeing whether it benefits you. If not, you can add riboflavin or feverfew, or the triple combination. Beyond these, the other supplements listed above are also worth trying, beginning perhaps with butterbur. I do recommend using 1–2 grams of fish oil per day from the start because the American Heart Association recommends this amount for preventing heart problems. The evidence for the importance of fish oils for preventing cardiovascular disease and death is irrefutable.

Nutrition and exercise are also important. Diet can sometimes play a major role in preventing migraines. Some foods are known to trigger migraines. These include alcohol, strong cheeses, avocados, vinegar, yogurt, sour cream, fermented (beer, wine) or cured foods, yeast products, nuts, chocolate, caffeine (including in nonprescription drugs or colas), and food additives (MSG, aspartame, nitrates). Many alternative physicians place patients on elimination diets to identify subtle food allergies.[25] Migraine sufferers also seem to do better when keeping a regular schedule of sleep and meals. Moderate exercise can also help, whereas intense exercise can sometimes be a trigger.

HOW MUCH MAGNESIUM TO TAKE

Due to the fact that people's responses to magnesium vary, I recommend starting at a lower dose than the recommended daily allowance (see page 26) and increasing gradually. For example, you might start by taking 100 milligrams of magnesium once or twice a day. Over a week or two, you can increase it to the RDA (320 milligrams for women, 420 milligrams for men). Whatever dosage you take, I recommend splitting it among two or three meals. It is best to take magnesium supplements with meals, as this improves absorption. Be sure to get plenty of fluids, because the body eliminates excess magnesium through the kidneys.

For medical conditions, people often have to use magnesium doses that are well above the RDA level. This should be done with medical supervision. If you are an older adult, have kidney impairment, or are taking drugs that can affect blood pressure, you should have your doctor supervise the use of magnesium. If magnesium causes gas or loose stools, refrain from use until it stops, then proceed again more gradually or switch to another type of magnesium supplement. It is not unusual to go through a little trial and error to find what works best for you. With long-term use, you should take calcium and other minerals in balance with the supplemental magnesium.

Unfortunately, getting your doctor's cooperation may be your greatest hurdle. Most doctors know little about magnesium. That is why I have written this book like an evidence-based medical journal article—the type of scientific paper that doctors respect. If you show your doctor this book and he or she still will not help, there are many other people you can turn to. Many other healthcare professionals—doctors who practice integrative medicine, nutritionists, naturopaths, nurses, chiropractors, and others—usually know about magnesium and can guide you.

Major problems with magnesium are rare. In 2000, an international journal stated, "The therapeutic window [the range of safe doses] of magnesium is wide, and in the absence of renal failure, severe side effects are extremely rare."[26] The rare case of magnesium toxicity that does arise usually occurs in a person with kidney impairments or in older people whose kidney functioning is reduced.

If you accidentally take more magnesium than your body can use or eliminate, the first symptoms you might experience include nausea, weakness, feeling of warmth, or flushing. Low blood pressure, reduced heart rate, double vision, and slurred speech can also occur. Like any mineral when taken at extremely high doses, severe magnesium toxicity can be dangerous; it can cause extreme weakness, vomiting, loss of reflexes, respiratory and/or cardiac arrest. Magnesium toxicity can be diagnosed by means of a blood test; total serum magnesium, which most medical laboratories perform, will reveal an elevated magnesium blood level. Magnesium toxicity is worsened by the presence of low calcium levels. Calcium gluconate is an effective antidote.

HOW TO USE MAGNESIUM SUCCESSFULLY

Using magnesium successfully depends on finding a product that agrees with you. Some people can take any product, but many people have difficulty with magnesium, especially cheap, low-quality products that are poorly absorbed. When you take magnesium tablets or capsules, your body absorbs only about 30 percent of the magnesium they contain. With many top-selling products, absorption is much less, as little as 10 percent. This is because minerals like magnesium—or calcium or iron—are the stuff of rocks, and the human body is not designed to absorb rocks. When magnesium is not absorbed, it goes to the colon and can cause gas or diarrhea. This is why Milk of Magnesia, which is intentionally formulated to be poorly absorbed, works very well as a laxative. Poor-quality magnesium supplements can have the same effect. Therefore, the type of magnesium you choose can be very important.

You cannot purchase magnesium in its pure form, because atomic magnesium, like most elements, has an electric charge and readily binds with other atoms in nature. That is why there are so many different types of magnesium supplements available: magnesium carbonate, magnesium oxide, magnesium chloride, magnesium sulfate, and others. For better absorption, some supplement companies combine magnesium with amino acids, producing magnesium maleate, magnesium citrate, magnesium lactate, or magnesium aspartate, which work well for many people.

When I developed erythromelalgia, I did not know much about magnesium, and I had great difficulty tolerating many magnesium supplements. My gut did not like any of them, not even the amino-acid complexes. I almost gave up, but finally found a type of magnesium that worked well: magnesium chelate, which is an organic complex of magnesium with amino acids and proteins. This is the type of magnesium I recommend for people who have trouble with other types of magnesium or who want to avoid the possibility of developing trouble. I also recommend magnesium chelate for people whose physicians recommend higher doses of magnesium for their medical conditions. Many vitamin and health food stores carry chelated magnesium supplements, or they can order some for you. You can also find many sources of magnesium chelate on the Internet.

My experience is that for people with vascular conditions, magnesium products that do not contain other minerals work better than combination formulas. Even for nutritional purposes, I prefer taking a separate magnesium supplement because many calcium-magnesium or other combination products contain poor-quality types of magnesium that are poorly absorbed.

If you have difficulty with magnesium pills, you may do better with a liquid solution, particularly magnesium chloride solution. Magnesium solutions cost more than tablets or capsules, but they are the best absorbed, best tolerated, and fastest acting forms of magnesium. Some vitamin and health food stores carry magnesium-only solutions or dissolvable powders, but these products tend to be hard to find on store shelves. However, stores can usually order liquid magnesium for you, or you can find it online. You can also find online another magnesium solution, magnesium citrate, which is probably the best type of solution. It is available from the offices of Dr. Billie Sahley and Dr. Sherry Rogers.

Overall, I prefer magnesium pills because they are

less expensive and more convenient to use than solutions, and their effects last longer throughout the day. But if you cannot tolerate them, a magnesium solution is for you. And because liquids are absorbed faster, a magnesium solution is ideal for acute vascular conditions such as acute migraines.

CONCLUSION

Twenty-five million people suffer migraine headaches, and millions more endure cluster headaches. These disorders are extremely painful, limit functioning, affect work performance, and reduce people's overall quality of life.

Seventy-five percent of the population is magnesium deficient. Most people are not aware of their magnesium deficiencies. Doctors routinely prescribe drugs for many conditions caused or worsened by magnesium deficiencies, but they rarely consider using magnesium itself. Multiple studies have linked magnesium deficiencies with migraines, and other studies demonstrate magnesium's effectiveness in treating migraine headaches, yet few doctors know anything about magnesium.

Instead, too many doctors turn too readily to powerful prescription drugs. Prescription medications can be very helpful, but they can also be harmful, are usually expensive, and do not address the underlying biochemical basis of disease. The fact is, many patients are not as enamored with the prescription drug approach as are their doctors. More than 25 percent of the prescriptions that doctors write are never filled. Patients fear side effects. Drug prices keep climbing. Furthermore, many patients feel that their doctors turn too quickly to drugs without giving any consideration to other, safer methods. Dr. Rogers, in *Tired or Toxic? A Blueprint for Health*, asserts: "Medicine is hooked on medicines. We need to get hooked on finding the bio-chemical deficits and correcting them."

I agree with her. For more than a decade, my research and publications have focused on how to pre-vent medication side effects while allowing people to get the treatment they need. Medications play an important role in healthcare, but they should not be the first choice in virtually every medical situation, as is the case in most doctors' offices today. As more and more nutritional therapies are discovered and proven effective, these safer, physiologically beneficial thera-pies must be integrated into the healthcare system. It is absurd that we have two medical systems today: main-stream and alternative. The only system that makes sense is an integrative medical system that incorpo-rates the best of both mainstream and alternative med-icine. You should not have to go to two different practitioners to get one complete picture. You should not have to go any further than your own doctor to learn about magnesium, and its role in normal vascu-lar functioning and in helping treat widespread vascu-lar disorders such as high blood pressure and migraine and cluster headaches.

Unfortunately, today's drug-oriented healthcare system is not very good at spreading the word about effective, non-drug methods. The big money is chan-neled into marketing and advertising expensive drugs to doctors and patients, which in turn produces big profits—and ever increasing healthcare and insurance costs. The result of our drug-oriented system is that doctors are not even aware of magnesium's vital role in preserving vascular function, preventing cardiac arrhythmias, reducing nerve excitability, or preventing or treating muscle cramps or spasms.

Magnesium is not a panacea. Magnesium can help millions, but it will not help everyone. Magnesium's benefits can occur quickly, but sometimes the benefits take time to build as the body works to move more magnesium into the cells. Some people respond to low or RDA doses of magnesium, whereas others need higher doses that should be taken under medical supervision.

All migraine sufferers should obtain a medical evaluation and proper diagnosis. If you have a migraine or cluster condition, foods and other triggers should be identified and avoided whenever possible. If treatment is necessary, magnesium is a natural element, easily available, safe, inexpensive, essential for normal body functioning—and proven to be highly effective for preventing and treating migraine and cluster headaches. If magnesium's benefits are not adequate, there are many other natural therapies you can try. Riboflavin (vitamin B_2) can be helpful, especially combined with magnesium. Fish oils and coenzyme Q_{10} are nutrients the body needs and effective for some migraine patients. Herbs such as feverfew and butterbur have been proven effective in clinical studies for reducing the frequency and severity of migraines. In addition, several companies make magnesium, riboflavin, and feverfew combinations that have helped thousands of people.

With the use of these therapies, relatively few people actually require prescription drugs for migraine or cluster headaches. If doctors knew about the effectiveness of these natural remedies, fewer drugs would be prescribed, fewer side effects would harm patients, and billions of dollars would be saved. I have written this book with two purposes: 1) to provide reliable information about magnesium and other natural therapies for migraine sufferers; and 2) to help get the word out about these non-drug therapies in order to shift doctors' emphasis from prescription drugs to an integrative approach. Medications have their role and can be a godsend, but medications should come last, not first. If the recommendations in this book are helpful for you, please help spread the word to your friends and your physicians.

REFERENCES

1. Magnesium, Migraines, and Cluster Headaches

1. Goadsby, P.J., Lipton, R.B., Ferrari, M.D. "Migraine—Current Understanding and Treatment." *New England Journal of Medicine*, 2002; 346(4):257–270.

2. Sacks, O. *Migraine*. University of California Press, Los Angeles: 1992.

3. Olesen, J., Tfelt-Hansen, P., Welch, K.M. *The Headaches*. Lippincott Williams and Wilkins, Philadelphia: 2000.

4. Davidoff, R. *Migraine: Manifestations, Pathogenesis, and Management*. F.A. Davis Company, Philadelphia: 1995.

5. Goadsby, P.J., Lipton, R.B., Ferrari, M.D. "Migraine—Current Understanding and Treatment." *New England Journal of Medicine*, 2002; 346(4):257–270.

6. *Ibid*.

7. *Ibid*.

8. Davidoff, R. *Migraine: Manifestations, Pathogenesis, and Management*. F.A. Davis Company, Philadelphia: 1995.

9. Latner, A.W. "34th Annual Top 200 Drugs." *Pharmacy Times*, 2000; 66(4):16–32.

10. Rude, R.D. "Magnesium deficiency: a cause of heterogeneous disease in humans." *Journal of Bone and Mineral Research*, 1998; 13(4):749–758.

11. Iseri, L.T., and French, J.H. "Magnesium: nature's physiologic calcium blocker." *American Heart Journal*, 1984; 108(1): 188–193.

12. Altura, B.M. "Calcium antagonist properties of magnesium: implications for antimigraine actions." *Magnesium*, 1985;4(4): 169–175.

13. Altura, Burton. Personal communication, Dec. 6, 2001.

14. Altura, B.M. "Calcium antagonist properties of magnesium: implications for antimigraine actions." *Magnesium*, 1985;4(4): 169–175.

15. Mauskop, A., Altura, B.M. "Role of magnesium in the pathogenesis and treatment of migraines." *Clinical Neuroscience*, 1998; 5(1):24–27.

16. Welch, K.M. "Current opinions in headache pathogenesis: introduction and synthesis." *Current Opinion in Neurology*, 1998; 11(3):193–197.

17. Rogers, S.A. *Tired or Toxic? A Blueprint for Health*. Prestige Publishing, Syracuse: 1990.

18. Rude, R.D. "Magnesium deficiency: a cause of heterogeneous disease in humans." *Journal of Bone and Mineral Research*, 1998; 13(4):749–758.

19. Rogers, S.A. *Tired or Toxic? A Blueprint for Health*. Prestige Publishing, Syracuse: 1990.

20. Whitaker, J. "Chapter 6: Miraculous Magnesium, Calcium, and Other Minerals Used Against Hypertension." In: *Dr. Whitaker's Hypertension Report—1997*.

21. Rogers, S.A. "Cure for Resistant Magnesium Deficiency." *Total Wellness Newsletter*, Nov. 2001:1–3.

22. "Eletriptan (Relpax) for migraine." *The Medical Letter On Drugs and Therapeutics*, 2003; 45:33–34.

23. Landy, S.H. "Migraine headaches and allodynia: early use of triptans to improve outcome." *Medscape*, Aug. 29, 2003: www.medscape.com/viewprogram/2617. Accessed 9/19/03.

24. *Physicians' Desk Reference*, 54th Edition. Montvale, NJ: Medical Economics Company, 2003.

25. *Ibid.*

26. Brandes, J.L., Saper, J.R., Diamond, M., et al. "Topiramate for migraine prevention." *JAMA*, 2004; 291:965–973.

27. *Physicians' Desk Reference*, 54th Edition. Montvale, NJ: Medical Economics Company, 2003.

28. Mueller L., Gallagher R.M., Ciervo, C.A. "Vasospasm-induced myocardial infarction with sumatriptan." *Headache*, 1996; 36(5): 32931.

29. Landy, S.H. "Migraine headaches and allodynia: early use of triptans to improve outcome." *Medscape*, Aug. 29, 2003: www.medscape.com/viewprogram/2617. Accessed 9/19/03.

30. *Physicians' Desk Reference*, 54th Edition. Montvale, NJ: Medical Economics Company, 2003.

31. Cady, R.K., et al. "The effect of magnesium on the responsiveness of migraineurs to a 5-HT1 agonist." *Neurology*, 1998; 50:A340.

32. Young, W.B., Hopkins, M.M., et al. "Topiramate: a case series study in migraine prophylaxis." *Cephalalgia*, 2002; 22:659-2D63.

33. Brandes, J.L., Saper, J.R., Diamond, M., et al. "Topiramate for migraine prevention." *JAMA*, 2004; 291:965–973.

34. Grady, D. "Quest for weight-loss drug takes an unusual turn." *New York Times*, Apr. 15, 2003: www.nytimes.com.

35. Brandes, J.L., Saper, J.R., Diamond, M., et al. "Topiramate for migraine prevention." *JAMA*, 2004; 291:965-973.

36. *Physicians' Desk Reference*, 54th Edition. Montvale, NJ: Medical Economics Company, 2003.

37. Wolfe, S.M., Editor. "Do not use for weight reduction: seizure medication topiramate (Topamax)." *Worst Pills, Best Pills News*, Public Citizen Health Research Group, Feb. 2004; 10:13–14.

38. *Ibid.*

39. Mauskop, A., Altura, B.T., Cracco, R.Q., and Altura, B.M. "Intravenous magnesium sulfate rapidly alleviates headaches of various types." *Headache*, 1996; 36(3):154–160.

40. Mauskop, A., and Fox, B. *What Your Doctor May Not Tell You About Migraines*. Warner Books, New York: 2001.

41. Rosenfeld, I. "Medical news that matters: Heads up, migraine sufferers." *Parade Magazine*, Jan. 5, 2003:19.

42. Brandes, J.L., Saper, J.R., Diamond, M., et al. "Topiramate for migraine prevention." *JAMA*, 2004; 291:965-973.

2. Magnesium Deficiency and Migraine Headaches

1. Altura, B.M. "Calcium antagonist properties of magnesium: implications for antimigraine actions." *Magnesium*, 1985;4(4):169–175.

2. Johnson, S. "The multifaceted and widespread pathology of magnesium deficiency." *Medical Hypotheses*, 2001; 56(2): 163–170.

3. Galan, P., et al. "Dietary magnesium intake in French adult population." In: Theophile, T., Anastassopoulou, J. *Magnesium: current status and new developments: theoretical, biological, and medical aspects.* Dordrecht [Netherlands]: Kluwer Academic, 1997.

4. Gaby, A. *Magnesium: How an Important Mineral Helps Prevent Heart Attacks and Relieve Stress.* Keats Publishing, New Canaan, CT: 1994.

5. Facchinetti, F., Sances, G., Borella, P., Genazzani, A.R., Nappi, G. "Magnesium prophylaxis of menstrual migraine: effects on intracellular magnesium." *Headache*, 1991; 31(5): 298–301.

6. Pfaffenrath, V., Wessely, P., Meyer, C., Isler, H.R., Evers, S., Grotemeyer, K.H. "Magnesium in the prophylaxis of migraine—a double-blind placebo-controlled study." *Cephalalgia*, 1996; 16(6): 436–440.

7. Peikert, A., Wilimzig, C., Kohne-Volland, R. "Prophylaxis of migraine with oral magnesium: results from a prospective, multicenter, placebo-controlled and double-blind randomized study." *Cephalalgia*, 1996; 16(4):257–263.

8. Mauskop, A., Altura, B.T., Cracco, R.Q., Altura, B.M. "Intra-

venous magnesium sulphate relieves migraine attacks in patients with low serum ionized magnesium levels: a pilot study." *Clinical Science*, 1995; 89(6):633–636.

9. Mauskop, A., Altura, B.T., Cracco, R.Q., and Altura, B.M. "Intravenous magnesium sulfate rapidly alleviates headaches of various types." *Headache*, 1996; 36(3):154–160.

10. Demirkaya, S., Vural, O., Dora, B., Topcuoglu, M.A. "Efficacy of intravenous magnesium sulfate in the treatment of acute migraine attacks." *Headache*, 2001; 41(2):171–177.

11. *Ibid*.

12. Mercola, J. "IV drugs or magnesium to treat migraine?" Optimal Illness Center website, Feb. 14, 2002: www.mercola. com.

13. Whang, R. "Chapter 2, Clinical Perturbations in Magnesium Metabolism." In: Theophile, T., and Anastassopoulou, J. *Magnesium: current status and new developments: theoretical, biological, and medical aspects*. Dordrecht [Netherlands]: Kluwer Academic, 1997.

14. Mende, C. Personal communication, Sept. 25, 2001.

15. Altura, B.M., and Altura, B.T. "Magnesium in Cardiovascular Biology." *Scientific American*, Science & Medicine, May/June 1995:28–37.

16. Marcus, J.C., Altura, B.T., and Altura, B.M. "Serum ionized magnesium in post-traumatic headaches." *Journal of Pediatrics*, 2001;139(3):459–462.

17. Mende, C. Personal communication, Sept. 25, 2001.

3. Magnesium Deficiencies in Migraine-Prone Populations

1. Warshaw, L.J., Lipton, R.B., Silberstein, S.D. "Migraine: a woman's disease." *Women and Health*, 1998; 28(2):79–99.

2. Olesen, J., Tfelt-Hansen, P., Welch, K.M. *The Headaches*. Lippincott Williams and Wilkins, Philadelphia: 2000.

3. Mende, C. Personal communication, Sept. 25, 2001.

4. Castelli, S., Meossi, C., Domenici, R., et al. "Magnesium in the prophylaxis of primary headache and other periodic disorders in children." *Pediatric Medical Chir*, 1993; 15(5): Abstract.

5. Wang, F., et al. "Oral magnesium oxide prophylaxis of frequent childhood migraine." *Cephalalgia*, 2000; 20:424.

6. Marcus, J.C., Altura, B.T., and Altura, B.M. "Serum ionized magnesium in post-traumatic headaches." *Journal of Pediatrics*, 2001;139(3):459–462.

7. Mauskop, A., Altura, B.T., Cracco, R.Q., Altura, B.M. "Serum ionized magnesium levels in patients with episodic and chronic cluster headaches." *Clinical Pharmacology and Therapeutics*, 1993; 53(2):227. Abstract.

8. Mauskop, A., Altura, B.T., Cracco, R.Q., and Altura, B.M. "Ionized magnesium, total magnesium, and ionized calcium ratios with episodic and chronic cluster headaches." *Headache Quarterly, Current Treatment and Research*, 1994; 5(2):156–158.

9. Mauskop, A., Altura, B.T., Cracco, R.Q., and Altura, B.M. "Intravenous magnesium sulfate relieves cluster headaches in patients with low serum ionized magnesium levels." *Headache*, 1995; 35(10):597–600.

4. How to Use Magnesium to Help Prevent and Treat Migraine and Cluster Headaches

1. Altura, Burton. Personal communication, Dec. 6, 2001.

2. Magaziner, A. Personal communications, Nov. 28, 2001 and Dec. 2, 2001.

3. Magaziner, A. Personal communications, Nov. 28, 2001 and Dec. 2, 2001.

4. Gaby, A. *Magnesium: How an Important Mineral Helps Prevent Heart Attacks and Relieve Stress.* Keats Publishing, New Canaan, CT: 1994.

5. Cohen, J.S. "High-Dose, Oral Magnesium in the Treatment of

Chronic, Intractable Erythromelalgia." *Annals of Pharmacotherapy*, Feb. 2002; 36:255–260.

6. Rogers, S.A. "Cure for Resistant Magnesium Deficiency." *Total Wellness Newsletter*, Nov. 2001:1–3.

7. Magaziner, A. Personal communications, Nov. 28, 2001 and Dec. 2, 2001.

8. Whitaker, J. "Minerals, Part 2: Miraculous Magnesium." *Health & Healing*, May 1999; 9(5):2.

9. Mende, C. Personal communication, Sept. 25, 2001.

10. Mauskop, A., and Fox, B. *What Your Doctor May Not Tell You About Migraines.* Warner Books, New York: 2001.

11. Schoenen, J., Lenaerts, M., and Bastings, E. "High-dose riboflavin as a prophylactic treatment of migraine." *Cephalalgia*, 1994; 14:328–329.

12. Schoenen, J., Jacquy, J., and Lenaerts, M. "Effectiveness of high-dose riboflavin in migraine prophylaxis." *Neurology*, 1998; 50: 466–470.

13. Fox, R. "Natural agents offer relief from the misery of migraines." *Life Extension*, Feb. 2004: 70–78.

14. Murphy, J.J., et al. "Randomized double-blind placebo-controlled trial of feverfew in migraine prevention." *Lancet*, 1988; 2:189–192.

15. Johnson, E.S., Kadam, N.P., et al. "Efficacy of feverfew as prophylactic treatment of migraine." *BMJ*, 1985; 291:569–573.

16. Fox, R. "Natural agents offer relief from the misery of migraines." *Life Extension*, Feb. 2004: 70–78.

17. *Ibid.*

18. *Ibid.*

19. Murphy, J.J., et al. "Randomized double-blind placebo-controlled trial of feverfew in migraine prevention." *Lancet*, 1988; 2:189–192.

20. Fox, R. "Natural agents offer relief from the misery of migraines." *Life Extension*, Feb. 2004: 70–78.

21. Mauskop, A., and Fox, B. *What Your Doctor May Not Tell You About Migraines.* Warner Books, New York: 2001.

22. "Evidence-based guidelines for migraine headache in the primary care setting." American Academy of Neurology, 2000.

23. Whitaker, J. "Migraines." Headache Resource. www. DrWhitaker.com, Dec. 3, 2001.

24. Gaby, A. *Magnesium: How an Important Mineral Helps Prevent Heart Attacks and Relieve Stress.* Keats Publishing, New Canaan, CT: 1994.

25. Monro, J., et al. "Migraine is a food allergic disease." *Lancet*, 1984; 2:719.

26. Saris, N.E., Mervaala, E., Karppanen, H., et al. "Magnesium: An update on physiological, clinical and analytical aspects." *Clinica Chimica Acta*, 2000; 294(1-2):1–26.

ABOUT THE AUTHOR

Dr. Jay Cohen is a widely recognized expert on prescription medications and non-drug alternatives that work. Dr. Cohen is an Associate Professor (voluntary) of Family and Preventive Medicine and of Psychiatry at the University of California, San Diego. Dr. Cohen graduated from Temple University School of Medicine in Philadelphia in 1971. After completing his internship, Dr. Cohen practiced general medicine, and then conducted pain research at UCLA. He then completed a psychiatry residency at the University of California, San Diego, and practiced psychiatry and psychopharmacology for thirteen years.

Since 1990, Dr. Cohen has been involved in clinical pharmacology, conducting independent research on medication side effects: why they occur and how they can be prevented. Dr. Cohen's research has identified multiple problems—in drug industry research, U.S. Food and Drug Administration review, and doctors' methods—that have contributed to medication side effects being the fourth leading cause of death in America. Dr. Cohen believes that most medication side effects are preventable.

Since 1996, Dr. Cohen has published his findings and solutions in leading medical journals including the *Archives of Internal Medicine, The Journal of the Amer-*

ican Medical Women's Association, Geriatrics, Drug Safety, and the *Annals of Pharmacotherapy.* He has also written articles for consumer publications such as *Newsweek, Bottom Line Health,* and *Life Extension Magazine.* His work has been featured in the *New York Times, Washington Post, Consumer Reports, Wall Street Journal, Modern Maturity, Women's Day,* and virtually every other major magazine and newspaper in America. His book, *Over Dose: The Case Against The Drug Companies* (Tarcher/ Putnam, Nov. 2001), received unanimously excellent reviews from *Publishers Weekly, Library Journal,* and others, as well as in the *Journal of the American Medical Association.*

Dr. Cohen practices preventive and anti-aging medicine that involves state-of-the-art analyses of metabolic, immune, hormonal, and other body systems as well as assessments of antioxidant, vitamin/mineral, essential fatty acid and other key functional capacities. Nutrition and natural supplements are then used in order to bring people into physiologic balance and to help slow the processes of degeneration and aging. Dr. Cohen also works with people who are sensitive to medications or who want to reduce or simplify their medication regimens. Areas of specialization include the non-drug treatment of high blood pressure, high cholesterol, migraine headaches, osteoporosis, and inflammatory conditions. Dr. Cohen's office is located in Del Mar, CA. For information, call 858-509-8944 or go to www.MedicationSense.com.

INDEX

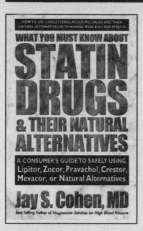

WHAT YOU MUST KNOW ABOUT STATIN DRUGS & THEIR NATURAL ALTERNATIVES

A Consumer's Guide to Safely Using Lipitor, Zocor, Pravachol, Crestor, Mevacor, or Natural Alternatives

Jay S. Cohen, MD

It is estimated that over 100 million Americans suffer from elevated cholesterol and C-reactive proteins—markers that are linked to heart attack, stroke, and other cardiovascular disorders. To combat these problems, modern science has created a group of drugs known either as statins or as specific commercial drugs such as Lipitor, Zocor, and Pravachol. While over 20 million people take these medications, the fact is that up to 42 percent experience side effects, and a whopping 60 to 75 percent eventually stop treatment. Here, for the first time, is a guide that explains the problems caused by statins, and offers easy-to-follow strategies that will allow you to benefit from these drugs while avoiding their side effects. In addition, the author discusses natural alternatives that have also proven effective.

What You Must Know About Statin Drugs & Their Natural Alternatives begins by explaining elevated cholesterol and C-reactive proteins. It then examines how statins work to alleviate these problems, and discusses possible side effects. Highlighted is information on safe usage, as well as a discussion of effective alternative treatments. If you have elevated cholesterol or C-reactive protein levels, or if you are currently using a statin, *What You Must Know About Statin Drugs & Their Natural Alternatives* can make a profound difference in the quality of your life.

$14.95 • 204 pages • 6 x 9-inch paperback • Health • ISBN 0-7570-0257-9

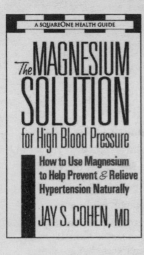

THE MAGNESIUM SOLUTION FOR HIGH BLOOD PRESSURE
How to Use Magnesium to Prevent and Relieve Hypertension Naturally

Jay S. Cohen, MD

More than 50 million Americans have high blood pressure—a devastating disease that can lead to heart attacks and strokes. Doctors routinely prescribe drugs for this condition, but these medications frequently cause side effects. As a nationally recognized expert on medications and side effects, Dr. Jay S. Cohen wants to make you aware of a safe, natural solution to high blood pressure—the mineral magnesium.

Magnesium is essential for the normal functioning of nerves, muscles, blood vessels, bones, and the heart, yet more than 75% of the population is deficient in it. Dr. Cohen has written *The Magnesium Solution for High Blood Pressure* to provide you and your doctor with all of the information needed to understand why magnesium is essential for helping to prevent and treat high blood pressure. Dr. Cohen explains why magnesium is necessary for normal vascular functioning, how to use magnesium along with hypertension drugs, and the best types of magnesium to use. Most importantly, Dr. Cohen has made the evidence-based research on magnesium's safety and effectiveness highly readable and usable by anyone.

$5.95 • 96 pages • 4 x 7-inch mass paperback • Health/Hypertension • ISBN 0-7570-0255-2